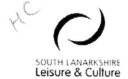

A BOOK ABOUT
DEPRESSION

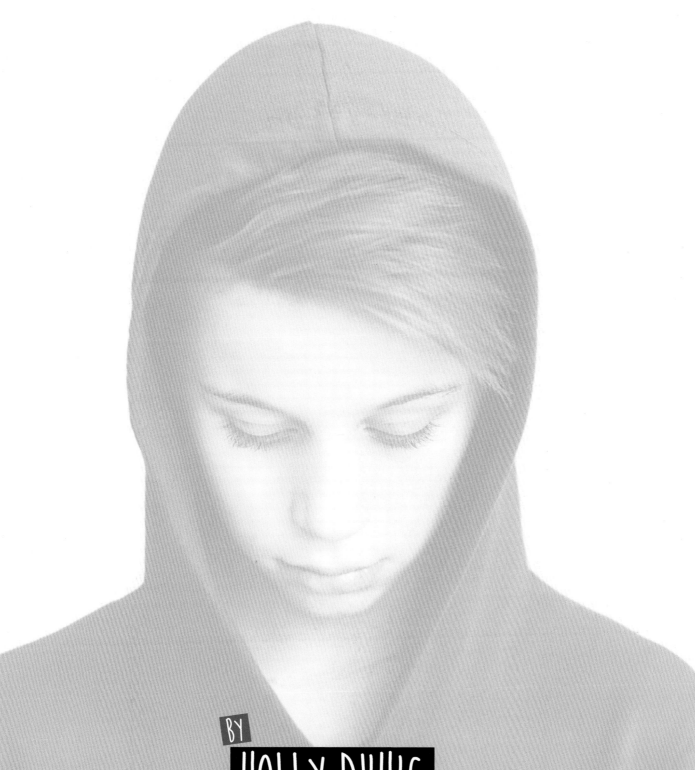

BY
HOLLY DUHIG

BookLife
PUBLISHING

©This edition published in
2022. First published in 2018.
BookLife Publishing Ltd.
King's Lynn, Norfolk
PE30 4LS, UK

A catalogue record for this
book is available from the
British Library.

ISBN: 978-1-78637-341-0

Written by:
Holly Duhig

Edited by:
Kirsty Holmes

Designed by:
Danielle Webster-Jones

With grateful thanks to Place2Be for their
endorsement of this series.

These titles have been developed to
support teachers and school counsellors
in exploring pupils' mental health, and
have been reviewed and approved by
the clinical team at Place2Be, the leading
national children's mental health charity.

PHOTO CREDITS

CONTENTS

Words that look like **THIS** are explained in the glossary on page 31.

WHAT IS DEPRESSION?

Depression is a mental health condition that causes people to feel very sad for a long period of time. Many people feel sad from time to time, for example when their favourite sports team loses a game, or when their friend moves to a new school. These feelings are not very nice, but they are **TEMPORARY** and will eventually go away.

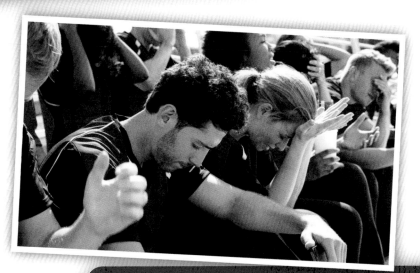

Feeling Sad Versus Feeling Depressed

Depression is similar to sadness, but it lasts longer and is a lot more **INTENSE** and complicated than simply being down in the dumps. Depression can cause feelings of hopelessness, low **MOTIVATION**, boredom and tearfulness, as well as sadness. Sometimes, people become depressed because of a specific event, such as a loved one passing away, but a lot of the time it is not caused by anything in particular. When you have depression, it can feel as if there's no hope of getting better, but it can be treated. Depression is usually treated with the help of a **THERAPIST**. Therapists are experts in treating mental health conditions and they can teach you all sorts of ways to cope with your feelings.

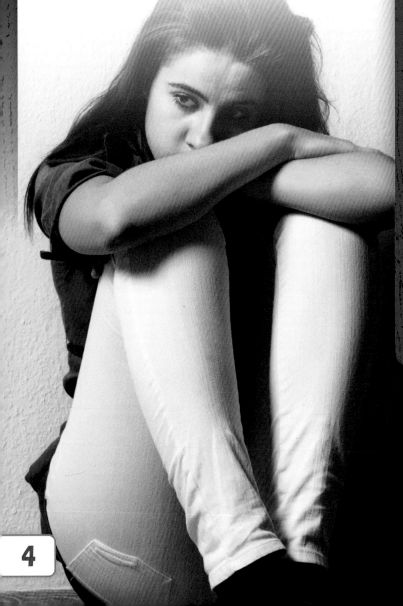

IN THE UK, ABOUT 17% OF PEOPLE AGED 5-16 ARE THOUGHT TO HAVE SOME KIND OF MENTAL HEALTH PROBLEM, INCLUDING DEPRESSION AND ANXIETY.

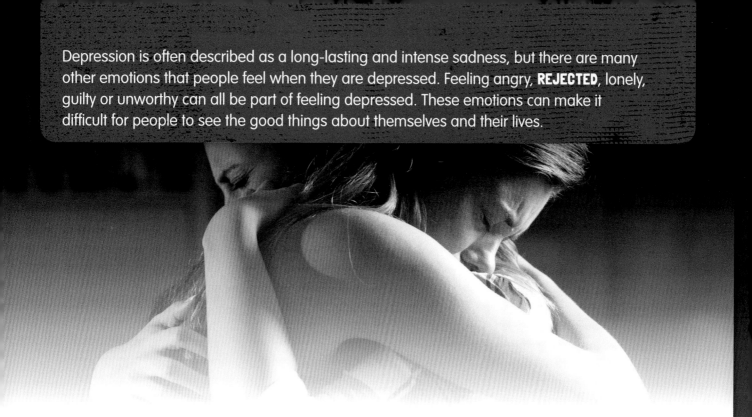

Depression is often described as a long-lasting and intense sadness, but there are many other emotions that people feel when they are depressed. Feeling angry, **REJECTED**, lonely, guilty or unworthy can all be part of feeling depressed. These emotions can make it difficult for people to see the good things about themselves and their lives.

People with depression are often told that simply thinking happier thoughts will help them feel less depressed. However, recovering from depression is not as easy as simply thinking happy thoughts. Depression is an illness and, like any other illnesses, it can take time to recover from it. What's more, depression actually makes it harder for people to think positive thoughts and experience positive emotions.

Many people are affected by depression at some point in their lives. Some people might experience one **PERIOD** of depression in their lifetime and then get better, while other people might experience depression many times throughout their lives. These people often take a type of medication, called an anti-depressant, to help them manage their depression.

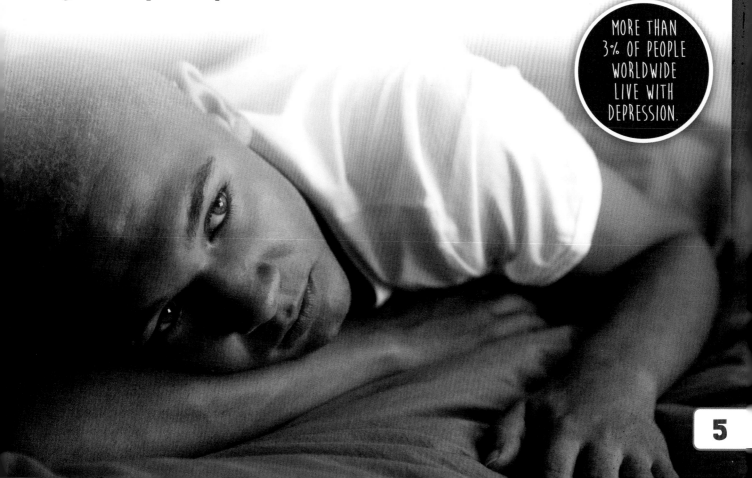

MORE THAN 3% OF PEOPLE WORLDWIDE LIVE WITH DEPRESSION.

SYMPTOMS OF DEPRESSION

Depression is a mood disorder, which means it mainly affects your mood and the way that you think and feel. However, it can also affect how you behave. For instance, many people with depression find themselves avoiding taking part in activities they used to enjoy. Some of the emotional symptoms of depression are:

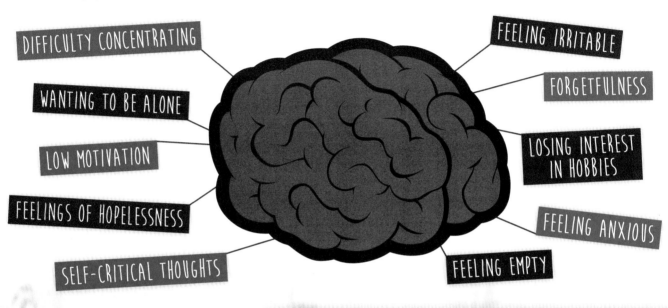

DIFFICULTY CONCENTRATING

WANTING TO BE ALONE

LOW MOTIVATION

FEELINGS OF HOPELESSNESS

SELF-CRITICAL THOUGHTS

FEELING IRRITABLE

FORGETFULNESS

LOSING INTEREST IN HOBBIES

FEELING ANXIOUS

FEELING EMPTY

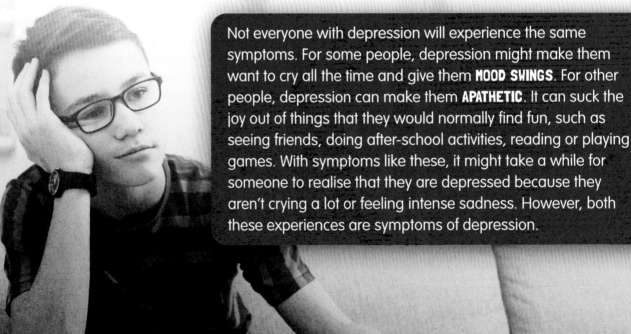

Not everyone with depression will experience the same symptoms. For some people, depression might make them want to cry all the time and give them **MOOD SWINGS**. For other people, depression can make them **APATHETIC**. It can suck the joy out of things that they would normally find fun, such as seeing friends, doing after-school activities, reading or playing games. With symptoms like these, it might take a while for someone to realise that they are depressed because they aren't crying a lot or feeling intense sadness. However, both these experiences are symptoms of depression.

Physical Symptoms of Depression

Many symptoms of depression affect our minds, but depression can also affect our bodies. Here are some of the **PHYSICAL** symptoms of depression:

Just as people can experience different emotional symptoms, people can also experience different physical symptoms. Some people with depression crave a lot of food while others don't want to eat at all. Scientists think that depression slows down the body's **DIGESTIVE SYSTEM**, which can cause people to feel unwell or need to go to the toilet more or less than usual. It can also cause people to lose their appetite and skip meals, which can make it even harder to cope with feelings of depression. This is because our brains use **GLUCOSE** from our food to work. When we don't eat enough, our brains can't get enough glucose. This affects our ability to manage our emotions as well as our ability to concentrate on everyday tasks.

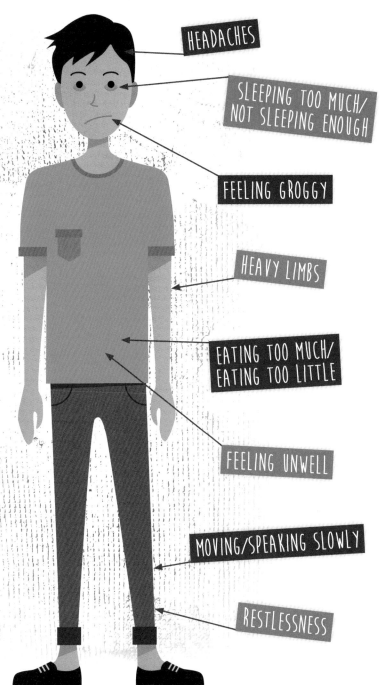

HEADACHES

SLEEPING TOO MUCH/ NOT SLEEPING ENOUGH

FEELING GROGGY

HEAVY LIMBS

EATING TOO MUCH/ EATING TOO LITTLE

FEELING UNWELL

MOVING/SPEAKING SLOWLY

RESTLESSNESS

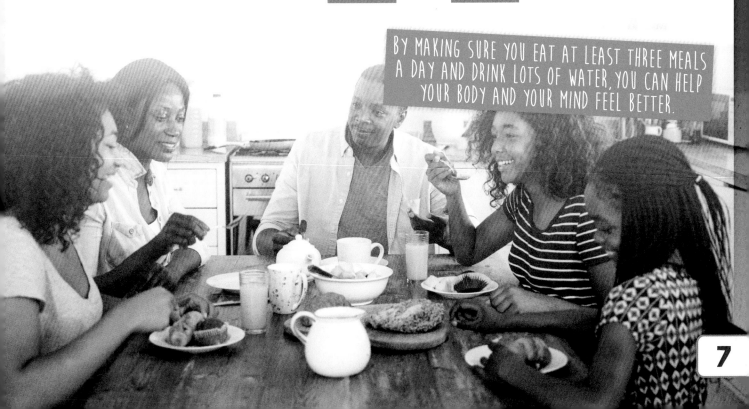

BY MAKING SURE YOU EAT AT LEAST THREE MEALS A DAY AND DRINK LOTS OF WATER, YOU CAN HELP YOUR BODY AND YOUR MIND FEEL BETTER.

AN INVISIBLE ILLNESS

Physical illnesses, such as chickenpox, have visible symptoms which show that you are unwell, such as spots or a rash. Mental health conditions, such as depression, often have very few visible signs that suggest you are unwell. Sometimes, the visible signs of depression will be mistaken for signs of feeling a bit tired or unwell. Because of this, people often don't see depression as an illness and think it can be easily overcome. This is not the case. Depression is an illness just like any other. However, depression is an illness that mostly affects the brain.

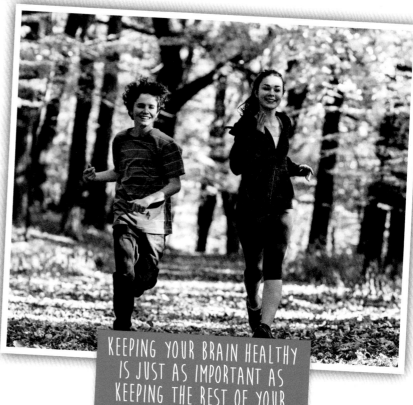

KEEPING YOUR BRAIN HEALTHY IS JUST AS IMPORTANT AS KEEPING THE REST OF YOUR BODY HEALTHY.

Some research has shown that certain parts of the brain are different in people with depression than in people without it. For example, the hippocampus, the part of the brain that deals with memory and emotion, has been seen to shrink in people who have gone through **SEVERE** depression. However, scientists have also found that it's possible for the hippocampus to grow again when someone recovers from depression by growing new brain cells.

HIPPOCAMPUS

DEPRESSION IS OFTEN CALLED AN INVISIBLE ILLNESS.

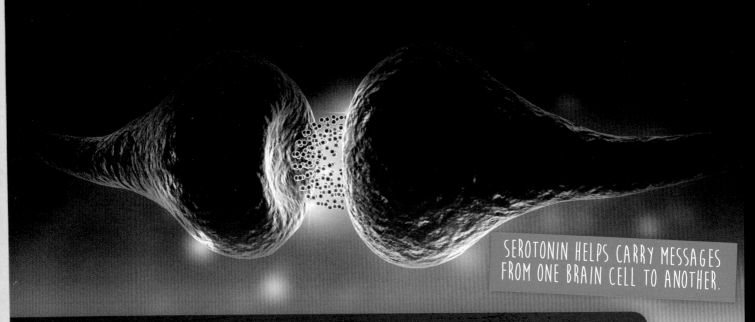

SEROTONIN HELPS CARRY MESSAGES FROM ONE BRAIN CELL TO ANOTHER.

The Science of Depression

Lots of scientific research has been done on the subject of depression in order to find out more about how it affects the brain and how it can be treated. Many scientists believe that depression is caused by an imbalance of **CHEMICALS** in the brain, especially chemicals that affect our moods. For example, some studies have shown that people who are depressed often have less of a chemical called serotonin, which sends messages around our brains and helps keep our moods stable. Some medications that doctors use to treat depression increase the amount of serotonin between brain cells.

Although scientists are trying really hard to find out exactly what causes depression, the truth is that no one knows for sure. Often, people become depressed because of a whole range of reasons. Some of these might be to do with someone's brain chemistry. However, depression might also happen due to unhappy life events and difficult experiences, such as losing a loved one, being bullied or growing up.

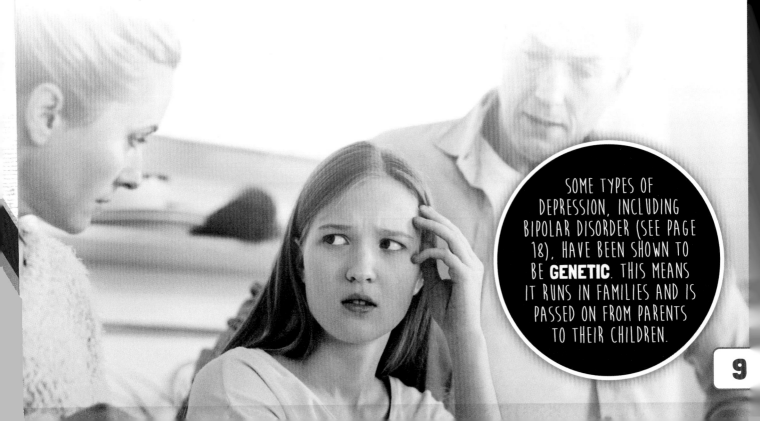

SOME TYPES OF DEPRESSION, INCLUDING BIPOLAR DISORDER (SEE PAGE 18), HAVE BEEN SHOWN TO BE **GENETIC**. THIS MEANS IT RUNS IN FAMILIES AND IS PASSED ON FROM PARENTS TO THEIR CHILDREN.

BODY IMAGE

Your body image is how you see your physical appearance, and it can have a big impact on your mood. Some people like what they see when they look in the mirror. This is called having a positive body image and is a very good thing. Other people don't like the way they look as much. This is called having a negative body image. For some people, their body image affects them so much that they become depressed.

There are lots of things that can affect our body image. As we get older, our bodies grow and change. The way we see our bodies might change as a result. We might also begin to compare ourselves to people we see in the **MEDIA** and online, such as celebrities, bloggers or our friends. However, it is important to remember that what we see on social media is often edited and doesn't show the true **DIVERSITY** of the way people look. If you start to change your eating habits or avoid certain activities because you are worried about the way you look, then it is time to talk to someone you trust about how you are feeling.

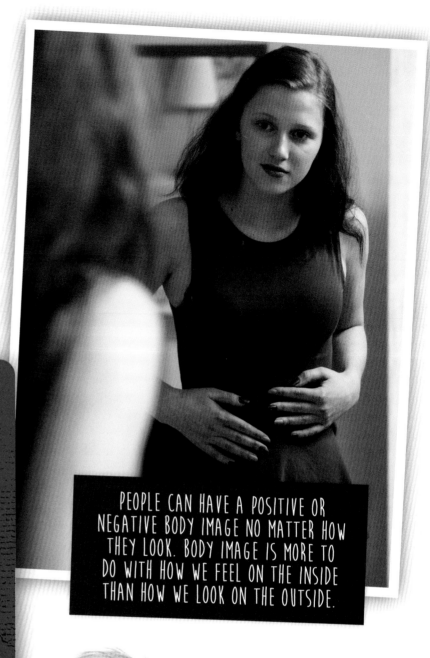

PEOPLE CAN HAVE A POSITIVE OR NEGATIVE BODY IMAGE NO MATTER HOW THEY LOOK. BODY IMAGE IS MORE TO DO WITH HOW WE FEEL ON THE INSIDE THAN HOW WE LOOK ON THE OUTSIDE.

KEEPING OUR BODIES AND OUR MINDS HEALTHY IS MUCH MORE IMPORTANT THAN THE WAY WE LOOK.

Grief

Sometimes people will experience a period of sadness after someone has died. This is called grief. Some people find that their grief lasts a very long time and becomes depression. It is also possible to feel OK for a while and then become depressed a long time after someone's death. This is usually a sign that you weren't able to deal with your feelings at the time, so they came out a bit later. The best thing to do is to talk to someone.

When someone close to you dies, it can be a very difficult thing to deal with. You might have a lot of different feelings, such as sadness, anger, guilt or loneliness. You might feel angry at friends, family or the world around you for letting bad things happen. You might even be angry at yourself or at the person who has died for leaving you. This is all perfectly normal and won't last forever. Grief can also make you feel very lonely and sad. You might cry a lot or feel empty inside. Grief usually lasts for a while and gets better over time.

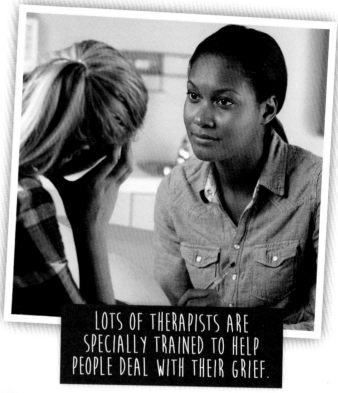

LOTS OF THERAPISTS ARE SPECIALLY TRAINED TO HELP PEOPLE DEAL WITH THEIR GRIEF.

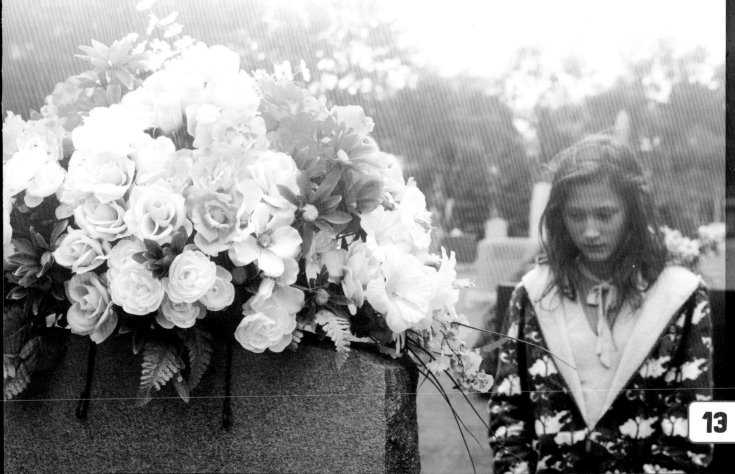

13

FEELING NUMB

Depression doesn't always happen for a reason. For some people, it just happens. This is because depression is an illness. Like a cough or a cold, anyone can experience it, no matter who they are or what their lives are like. There doesn't have to be a reason for someone to be depressed. Lots of adults and children with depression are told that they have 'no reason' to feel down because there are other people in worse situations than them. This is not helpful. It can make people feel guilty about being depressed, which can then make their depression even worse. People can't help their feelings and there is no way that we 'should' feel. It is OK not to always feel OK.

IF A PARENT OR CARER IS DEPRESSED, JUST SHOWING THAT YOU ARE THERE FOR THEM CAN HELP. IF YOU FEEL ALONE, TELL SOMEONE. TALK TO ANOTHER CAREGIVER OR FAMILY MEMBER IF YOU CAN.

Depression is often talked about as a deep sadness, but a lot of the time depression just feels like nothing. It can make you feel **NUMB**, which makes it hard to care about anything at all. For people with loved ones and family members who are going through depression, this can be tricky to understand. It might feel like your loved one doesn't care about you anymore, but this is not the case. Sometimes, people with depression have been caring so much for so long that they can no longer express those feelings. It's like their brain is on standby mode.

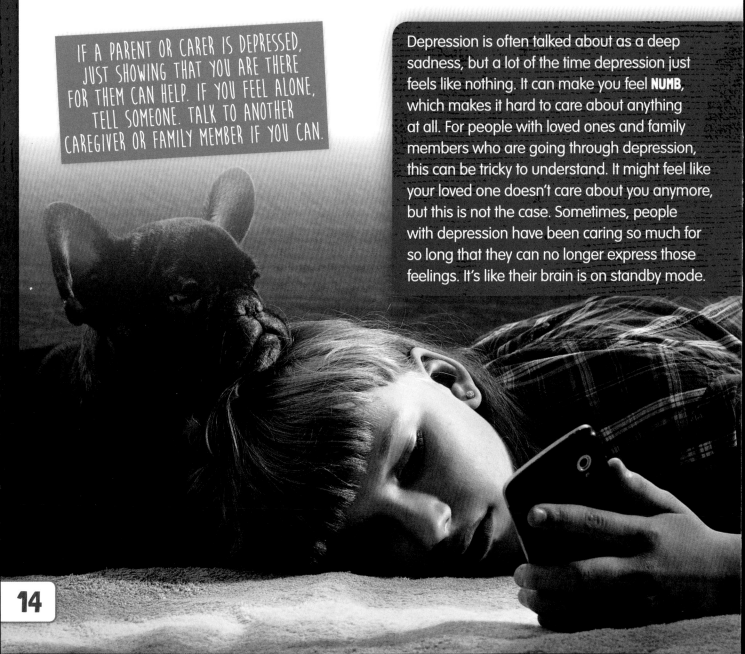

Depression can feel like having a foggy mind, where even the smallest things, such as getting something to eat or having a bath, feel tiring and pointless. When even small tasks are hard to do, more important things, such as asking for help, also feel pointless.

It is never pointless to ask for help, and there are lots of ways to do it. Here are just a few:

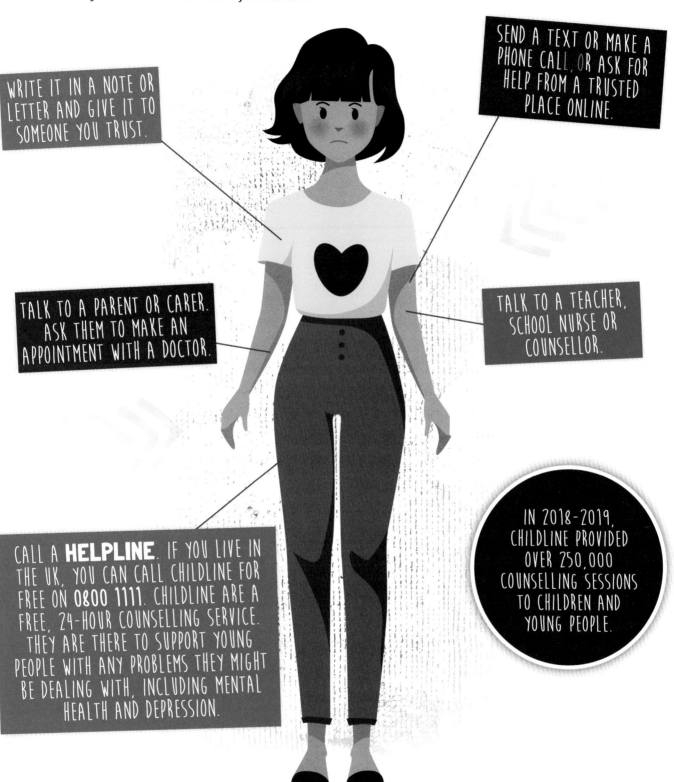

WRITE IT IN A NOTE OR LETTER AND GIVE IT TO SOMEONE YOU TRUST.

SEND A TEXT OR MAKE A PHONE CALL, OR ASK FOR HELP FROM A TRUSTED PLACE ONLINE.

TALK TO A PARENT OR CARER. ASK THEM TO MAKE AN APPOINTMENT WITH A DOCTOR.

TALK TO A TEACHER, SCHOOL NURSE OR COUNSELLOR.

CALL A **HELPLINE**. IF YOU LIVE IN THE UK, YOU CAN CALL CHILDLINE FOR FREE ON 0800 1111. CHILDLINE ARE A FREE, 24-HOUR COUNSELLING SERVICE. THEY ARE THERE TO SUPPORT YOUNG PEOPLE WITH ANY PROBLEMS THEY MIGHT BE DEALING WITH, INCLUDING MENTAL HEALTH AND DEPRESSION.

IN 2018-2019, CHILDLINE PROVIDED OVER 250,000 COUNSELLING SESSIONS TO CHILDREN AND YOUNG PEOPLE.

EVEN IF IT DOESN'T SEEM LIKE IT NOW, YOUR HEALTH AND WELL-BEING IS IMPORTANT. ASKING FOR HELP IS NEVER POINTLESS.

15

CASE STUDY: MEGAN

My name is Megan. Last year, my grandma passed away really suddenly. She used to live next door to our house, so I went there all the time and helped her cook dinner. When she died, I was extremely upset and I cried a lot. Mum tried to help me feel better, but she was upset too, because my grandma was her mum.

After Grandma's funeral, I didn't cry as much anymore, but I still didn't feel like myself. After a few months, I started thinking about Grandma less and less, but I still felt sad. It felt like there was something heavy on my shoulders weighing me down and all I wanted to do was lie on my bed. I just wanted to be left alone. I didn't really feel hungry for lunches and dinners anymore. It wasn't the same if they weren't cooked by Grandma.

At school, everything felt like too much. The work made my head fuzzy and I didn't see the point in getting good marks anymore. I got lots of headaches and had to see the school nurse a lot.

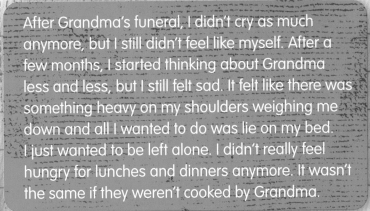

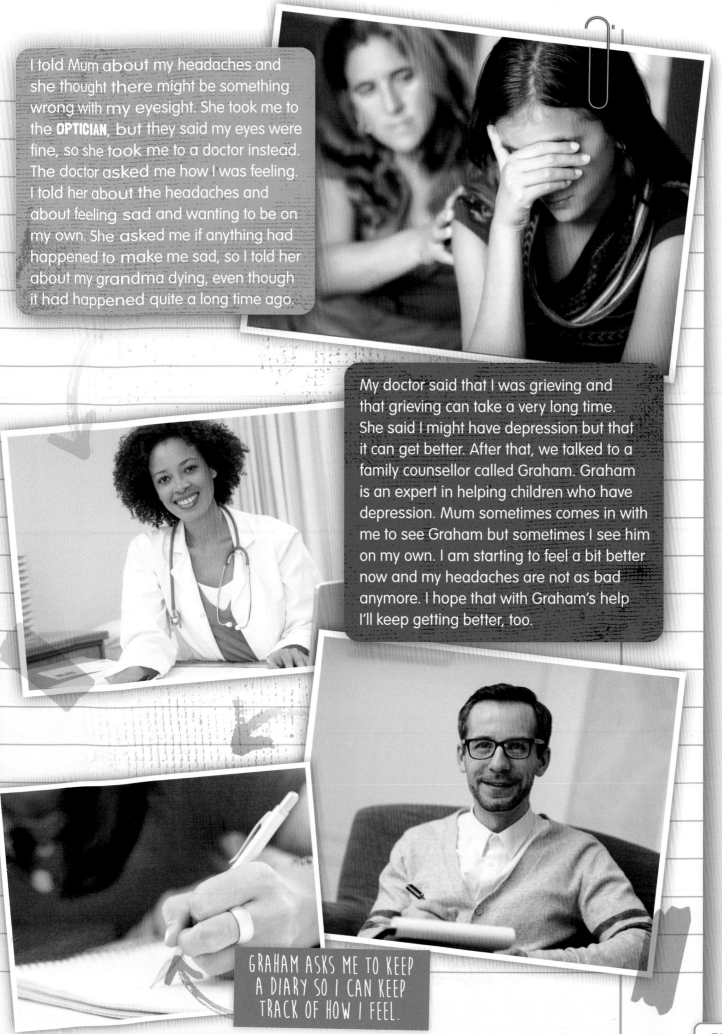

I told Mum about my headaches and she thought there might be something wrong with my eyesight. She took me to the **OPTICIAN**, but they said my eyes were fine, so she took me to a doctor instead. The doctor asked me how I was feeling. I told her about the headaches and about feeling sad and wanting to be on my own. She asked me if anything had happened to make me sad, so I told her about my grandma dying, even though it had happened quite a long time ago.

My doctor said that I was grieving and that grieving can take a very long time. She said I might have depression but that it can get better. After that, we talked to a family counsellor called Graham. Graham is an expert in helping children who have depression. Mum sometimes comes in with me to see Graham but sometimes I see him on my own. I am starting to feel a bit better now and my headaches are not as bad anymore. I hope that with Graham's help I'll keep getting better, too.

GRAHAM ASKS ME TO KEEP A DIARY SO I CAN KEEP TRACK OF HOW I FEEL.

VISUALISATION AND
MINDFULNESS

When we are depressed, it can feel like everything around us is going wrong or is bad in some way. One way to demonstrate how your brain works when you're depressed is to practice these steps.

STEP 1:

START BY CLOSING YOUR EYES AND **VISUALISING** THE ROOM AROUND YOU. WHILE YOUR EYES ARE CLOSED, TRY TO REMEMBER ALL OF THE OBJECTS IN THE ROOM THAT ARE RED. TRY NOT TO LOOK AROUND TOO MUCH BEFORE YOU CLOSE YOUR EYES! WHEN YOU OPEN YOUR EYES AGAIN, YOU WILL AUTOMATICALLY FOCUS ON ALL THE THINGS THAT ARE RED. THIS IS A BIT LIKE WHAT HAPPENS IN YOUR MIND WHEN YOU HAVE DEPRESSION. WHEN YOU ARE FEELING EXTREMELY SAD AND YOUR THOUGHTS ARE VERY NEGATIVE, YOU WILL AUTOMATICALLY PAY ATTENTION TO NEGATIVE THINGS IN THE WORLD AROUND YOU.

STEP 2:

YOU WILL PROBABLY START TO NOTICE LOTS OF RED OBJECTS THAT YOU DIDN'T SEE BEFORE. NOW, EACH TIME YOU SPOT A RED OBJECT, TRY TO VISUALISE SOMETHING GOOD. IT COULD BE SOMEONE YOU LOVE, A KIND THOUGHT ABOUT YOURSELF OR EVEN A GOOD THING THAT HAPPENED RECENTLY. OVER TIME, BY USING THIS TECHNIQUE, YOU MAY BE ABLE TO CHANGE SOME OF YOUR THOUGHT PATTERNS INTO MORE POSITIVE THOUGHT PATTERNS.

Snow Globe Visualisation

Mindfulness is the practice of focusing on the present, instead of worrying about the future or dwelling on the past, in order to feel more relaxed and positive. If you are feeling depressed or anxious, it can sometimes feel like there's a storm going on in your mind. Mindfulness uses visualisation to help calm your mind and your body at the same time.

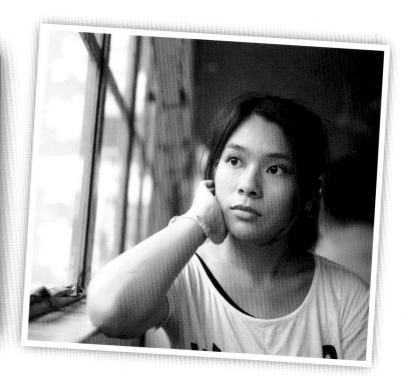

STEP 1:

CLOSE YOUR EYES AND VISUALISE SHAKING A SNOW GLOBE. TRY TO PICTURE THE SWIRLING SNOW SURROUNDING THE LITTLE HOUSE IN THE MIDDLE. IT IS NOT A VERY CALM SCENE. NOW TAKE A DEEP BREATH IN AND OUT AND VISUALISE HOLDING THE SNOW GLOBE STILL IN THE PALM OF YOUR HAND.

STEP 2:

AS YOU DO THIS, PAY ATTENTION TO THE MUSCLES IN YOUR BODY AND TRY TO KEEP THEM AS STILL AND RELAXED AS POSSIBLE. IMAGINE THE SNOW DRIFTING SLOWLY TO THE BOTTOM OF THE SNOW GLOBE AS YOU RELAX EACH MUSCLE IN YOUR BODY. THIS IS A MUCH CALMER SCENE.

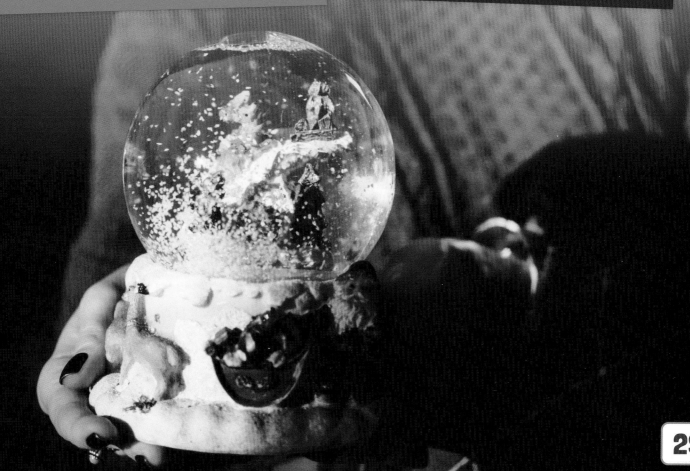

DEPRESSION

Even though there is now much more awareness of mental health conditions such as depression and how they affect people, many people still feel like they can't talk openly about their feelings. Keeping quiet about depression creates **STIGMA** and can make people who have depression feel very alone. It is important to remember that having depression does not make you weak or faulty in any way. In fact, depression takes a lot of strength to fight and people with depression are very brave.

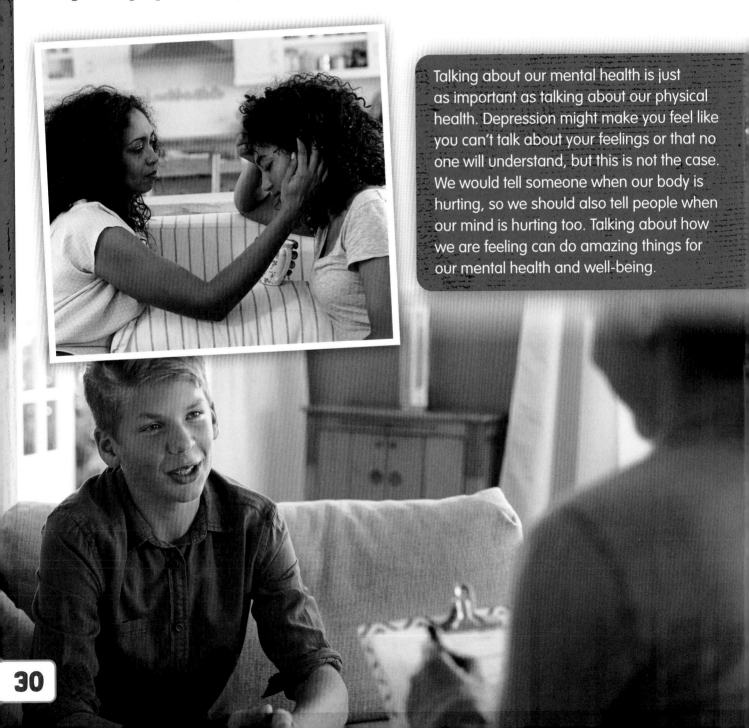

Talking about our mental health is just as important as talking about our physical health. Depression might make you feel like you can't talk about your feelings or that no one will understand, but this is not the case. We would tell someone when our body is hurting, so we should also tell people when our mind is hurting too. Talking about how we are feeling can do amazing things for our mental health and well-being.

GLOSSARY

APATHETIC	showing or feeling no interest, enthusiasm, or concern
AUTOMATIC	without using thought or control to do something
CHEMICALS	things made in the body that can cause changes to happen to it
DIGESTIVE SYSTEM	a group of body parts that break down food into things that can be taken in and used for energy
DISTORTED	misleading or false
DIVERSITY	a variety
EVIDENCE	the available facts or information used to prove whether or not something is true
EXAGGERATED	made to seem bigger, better or worse than it really is
GENETIC	something passed from a parent to their children via genes
GLUCOSE	a type of sugar that is an important way for living things to get energy
HELPLINE	a telephone service that provides help for people in need
INTENSE	to a strong amount
MEDIA	a way of sharing information with lots of people through things such as magazines, newspapers, television, radio and the internet
MOOD SWINGS	quick and dramatic changes in the way we feel
MOTIVATION	feeling like you want to do something
NUMB	the lack of feeling in your body or emotions
OPTICIAN	a person whose job it is to find problems with the eyes
PERIOD	a length of time
PHYSICAL	relating to the body
REJECTED	not cared about or given attention
SEVERE	(of something bad) serious, very great or in a strong way
SOLITARY	done or existing alone
STIGMA	a set of negative and often unfair beliefs about something
TEMPORARY	only lasting for a short time
THERAPIST	a person who is specially trained to treat mental health conditions
VERBALLY	by using words
VISUALISING	imagining as if something was real

INDEX